Gluten-Free Food List

Fueling Your Body, Nourishing Your Soul:
Balancing Nutrition and Flavor in
Gluten-Free Eating

McDonnell B. Young

Table of Contents

Introduction

Sarah Thompson stood in the middle of the bustling grocery store, her shopping cart empty despite the aisles bursting with options. Her recent diagnosis of celiac disease had turned what used to be a mundane task into a daunting challenge. Gluten, a protein she had barely thought about before, was now her nemesis, hiding in countless foods that had once filled her pantry.

It was during one such overwhelming grocery trip that Sarah stumbled upon a guide titled "Gluten-Free Food List: Your Comprehensive Guide to Safe Eating." At first, she was skeptical—after all, how many times had she come home with products that promised safety only to suffer the consequences later? But desperation and curiosity won over, and she decided to give the guide a chance.

The guide was divided thoughtfully into detailed chapters, the first of which explained what gluten was and its impact on those with celiac disease or gluten sensitivity. It provided comfort to Sarah, knowing she was not alone in her struggle and that her dietary changes were both necessary and beneficial.

As Sarah delved deeper, she found a comprehensive list of safe foods, neatly categorized into fruits, vegetables, proteins, and more. Each section was detailed and informative, teaching her not only what to eat but also how to identify hidden sources of gluten in processed foods and condiments.

The chapter on foods to avoid was an eye-opener. It listed not just the obvious foods like bread and pasta, but also lesser-known culprits like certain soups, sauces, and even some medications. The guide also included a segment on how to read labels effectively, a skill Sarah realized she sorely needed.

Equipped with her new guide, Sarah's trips to the grocery store transformed from stressful to empowering. She now knew which sections to visit and what brands to trust, saving her both time and the risk of accidental gluten ingestion. The guide even had tips for dining out and attending social events, areas of her life that had become sources of anxiety.

Months passed, and Sarah's health improved drastically. Grateful for the changes, she recommended the guide to online support groups and local celiac disease associations, sharing how it had educated and liberated her in managing her diet.

The guide was more than just a list; it was a tool that helped her regain control over her health and her life. It had comprehensive meal planning tips and gluten-free recipes that diversified her diet without compromising on taste or nutrition. Sarah felt equipped not just to live gluten-free, but to thrive.

One sunny afternoon, as Sarah hosted a gluten-free barbecue for friends and family, she reflected on her journey. Her guests, many of whom were not gluten-sensitive, marveled at the delicious and diverse foods on offer, all prepared safely according to her guide.

"To think, all this started with a little guidebook," Sarah mused, serving up grilled gluten-free pizzas and fresh salads. The guide hadn't just changed her diet; it had expanded her community and brought her joy in sharing her new, safe culinary discoveries.

As the laughter and conversation flowed around her garden, Sarah knew that recommending the "Gluten-Free Food List" guide was not just about listing safe foods—it was about offering hope and practical solutions to those feeling lost in their gluten-free journey, just as she once had.

Understanding Gluten: What It Is and Why It Matters

Gluten is a protein composite found in wheat, barley, rye, and triticale—a cross between wheat and rye. It acts as a glue that holds food together, helping it maintain its shape and can be found in a variety of products, from the obvious bread and pastries to less apparent foods like sauces and processed snacks. For many, gluten is harmless, but for others, it poses significant health challenges. Understanding the nature of gluten and its effects on the body is crucial for those needing or choosing to follow a gluten-free diet.

The primary reason gluten matters so much is due to celiac disease, an autoimmune disorder where the ingestion of gluten leads to damage in the small intestine. When people with celiac disease consume gluten, their immune system mounts an attack on the intestine, impairing nutrient absorption and leading to a host of complications ranging from abdominal pain and bloating to long-term intestinal damage and nutritional deficiencies. The only effective treatment for celiac disease is a strict, lifelong gluten-free diet.

Beyond celiac disease, some individuals experience non-celiac gluten sensitivity. This condition is marked by symptoms similar to celiac disease, including foggy mind, depression, abdominal pain, diarrhea, headaches, bone or joint pain, and chronic fatigue when gluten is consumed. Unlike celiac disease, non-celiac gluten sensitivity does not damage the small intestine. Still, a gluten-free diet is recommended to alleviate symptoms, which can significantly impact quality of life.

Another condition related to gluten is wheat allergy, which is an allergic reaction to proteins found in wheat, including gluten. Symptoms can include itching, swelling of the mouth or throat, difficulty breathing, and anaphylaxis, which can be life-threatening. Avoidance of wheat and wheat products is essential for managing this allergy.

The rise in popularity of gluten-free diets has also seen individuals without specific medical conditions opting to avoid gluten. Some claim that a gluten-free lifestyle leads to increased energy, weight loss, and a generally healthier lifestyle, although these benefits are not universally supported by scientific evidence. However, for those without an underlying health condition, the necessity of a gluten-free diet remains debatable, and nutritionists often warn against the risk of missing out on essential nutrients found in whole grains containing gluten.

Navigating a gluten-free diet can be challenging due to the widespread use of gluten in food products. Gluten is often used as a stabilizing agent in products like ice cream and ketchup, and can be found in bulk foods due to cross-contamination. This widespread use makes understanding food labels and ingredients critical for those following a gluten-free diet. Manufacturers are increasingly acknowledging the needs of gluten-sensitive consumers, and more products are being marketed as gluten-free, making it somewhat easier to maintain this diet.

In summary, gluten plays a significant role in various dietary conditions, influencing the health and wellbeing of many individuals. Whether due to celiac disease, gluten sensitivity, or personal choice, understanding gluten and its potential effects is essential for managing health through diet. As awareness and understanding grow, so does the availability of gluten-free options, making adherence to a gluten-free diet more manageable and helping those affected avoid the complications associated with gluten consumption.

Who Should Follow a Gluten-Free Diet?

A gluten-free diet is essential for individuals diagnosed with celiac disease, an autoimmune disorder where the ingestion of gluten leads to damage in the small intestine. When people with celiac disease consume gluten—a protein found in wheat, barley, and rye—their body mounts an immune response that attacks the small intestine. This can lead to symptoms like diarrhea, fatigue, and bloating, and over time, impede the absorption of nutrients, potentially causing a range of health issues from anemia to osteoporosis.

Beyond celiac disease, the diet is also recommended for those with non-celiac gluten sensitivity. This condition elicits similar symptoms to celiac disease when gluten is consumed, but unlike celiac, it does not cause lasting harm to the body's tissues. Symptoms can be varied and include gastrointestinal problems as well as joint pain, headaches, and fatigue. The only way to manage these symptoms is through a strict gluten-free diet, even though the sensitivity does not cause permanent gut damage.

Dermatitis herpetiformis, often termed as celiac disease's "skin manifestation," is another condition requiring a gluten-free diet. This chronic skin condition is characterized by itchy, blistering skin, and is directly linked to gluten ingestion. A gluten-free diet not only helps to control the outbreaks but is also necessary to prevent further complications associated with the underlying celiac disease.

Some people with wheat allergy may also benefit from a gluten-free diet, though in this case, they must avoid wheat specifically. Wheat allergy is different from celiac disease and gluten sensitivity because it is a classic food allergy involving a different immune response. While avoiding wheat, individuals with wheat allergies might tolerate other gluten-containing grains; however, many find it easier to adopt a fully gluten-free diet to ensure safety.

Moreover, individuals diagnosed with certain other autoimmune disorders, such as type 1 diabetes, thyroid diseases, and autoimmune liver diseases, may find improvement in their symptoms with a gluten-free diet. Research suggests that these conditions can have overlapping genetic markers with celiac disease, and dietary changes can sometimes mitigate immune responses.

A gluten-free diet is also being explored for its benefits in reducing symptoms of other conditions like irritable bowel syndrome (IBS) and attention deficit hyperactivity disorder (ADHD). Although the evidence is not conclusive, some patients report symptom relief after removing gluten from their diets, possibly due to a reduction in overall inflammation or a placebo effect.

While a gluten-free diet can be beneficial for various health conditions, it is crucial to approach this dietary change under medical guidance. Misguided self-diagnosis can lead to overlooking other health issues or nutrient deficiencies. Anyone considering a gluten-free diet should consult healthcare professionals to ensure a balanced diet and effective management of their specific health needs. This approach ensures that the diet is not only followed for appropriate reasons but also managed in a way that maintains overall nutritional health.

Benefits of Going Gluten-Free

Going gluten-free has been a transformative health decision for many, particularly for those with celiac disease or gluten sensitivity. For these individuals, eliminating gluten from their diet is not a choice but a necessity. Beyond this, even individuals without specific gluten-related disorders are discovering potential health benefits from adopting a gluten-free lifestyle. This includes improved digestive health, as removing gluten can alleviate symptoms like bloating, gas, diarrhea, and even constipation in some sensitive individuals. The improvement in digestive symptoms often leads to better absorption of essential nutrients, promoting overall health.

One of the less discussed benefits of a gluten-free diet is the potential for enhanced mental clarity and a reduction in fatigue. Some people report feeling less "foggy" and more energetic after removing gluten from their diets. This could be linked to a decrease in inflammation typically caused by gluten in sensitive individuals, which can impact brain function and energy levels. The diet also encourages the consumption of more whole and unprocessed foods such as fruits, vegetables, and lean proteins, which are naturally richer in the nutrients that promote brain health.

Weight management is another area where a gluten-free diet can make a significant impact. Although not inherently a weight loss diet, the elimination of many high-calorie, processed foods that contain gluten might help some people reduce their calorie intake naturally. Foods such as cakes, cookies, and pastas are replaced with whole grains like quinoa and other nutrient-dense alternatives, leading to a more balanced diet. This can help with better weight control and a healthier approach to eating overall.

People with autoimmune diseases other than celiac disease, like rheumatoid arthritis, have also seen improvements on a gluten-free diet. The reduction in systemic inflammation that can result from a gluten-free diet might help alleviate the painful symptoms associated with these conditions. Although research is still evolving in this area, the anecdotal evidence from those who have seen improvements is compelling.

The diet also promotes a greater awareness of food ingredients, encouraging individuals to choose more health-conscious options. This increased awareness can lead to a healthier overall diet that limits processed foods and includes more natural, unprocessed foods. As a result, individuals often experience an overall improvement in their health by following a diet that supports their body's needs without the added irritants and harmful ingredients.

For those concerned about allergic reactions and intolerances, a gluten-free diet offers a clear path to avoiding the discomfort and health issues associated with these conditions. Gluten can be a major irritant for many, and its removal from the diet can significantly improve quality of life for those with gluten-related disorders. This is especially important for children and adults who may face developmental and health challenges due to undiagnosed sensitivities or allergies.

Finally, the gluten-free diet's popularity has spurred a significant increase in the availability and variety of gluten-free products. Consumers now have access to a wide array of gluten-free alternatives that were not available in the past, making it easier to adhere to the diet without feeling deprived. This accessibility helps people sustain a gluten-free lifestyle long-term, contributing to continued health benefits and a better quality of life.

Reading Labels: Identifying Hidden Gluten

When shopping for gluten-free products, the ability to read and understand food labels is crucial. Gluten, a protein found in wheat, barley, and rye, can appear in many forms and under numerous names that might not be immediately recognizable. For those with celiac disease or gluten sensitivity, ingesting even a small amount of gluten can lead to serious health consequences, making vigilance essential.

One of the first steps in identifying hidden gluten on food labels is to look for obvious mentions of wheat, barley, rye, and triticale. These will often be highlighted as they are common allergens, but the presence of gluten can be less apparent in other ingredients. For example, malt, which is typically derived from barley, is a frequent additive in processed foods and can be listed as malt flavoring, malt extract, or malt syrup.

Beyond these direct mentions, it's important to be wary of terms like 'starch' or 'food starch.' While these can sometimes refer to cornstarch or another gluten-free starch, unless explicitly labeled as such, they often derive from wheat. Similarly, 'hydrolyzed vegetable protein' is another ingredient to approach with caution, as it can be sourced from wheat unless otherwise stated.

Other less obvious sources of gluten include dextrin, an additive sometimes sourced from wheat starch, and texturized vegetable protein, which often contains gluten unless specifically noted otherwise. Even natural flavorings and seasonings can be suspect, as they may contain gluten without clear labeling. In such cases, contacting the manufacturer to confirm the source of these ambiguous ingredients can be a necessary step for those who need to avoid gluten strictly.

In addition to knowing what to look for, understanding certification and labeling laws can also assist consumers. In many regions, foods labeled as 'gluten-free' must meet strict standards, generally containing less than 20 parts per million of gluten. However, products labeled as 'no gluten,' 'free of gluten,' and 'without gluten' are not regulated in the same way and may not meet these stringent requirements.

Another helpful tip is to utilize technology and resources tailored to the gluten-free community. Many smartphone apps and websites specialize in identifying products and brands that are safe for those with gluten sensitivities. These resources often provide user reviews and up-to-date research about new products on the market, which can be incredibly helpful.

Ultimately, becoming proficient in reading labels for hidden gluten requires continuous learning and attention to detail. As manufacturers frequently change their recipes or the sources of their ingredients, maintaining a current knowledge base is vital. Engaging with online communities, staying informed through credible gluten-free advocacy groups, and regularly reviewing updated materials on gluten-free living are all effective strategies for managing a gluten-free diet safely and effectively.

Chapter 1: Gluten-Free Foods

Fruits and Vegetables

Here's a detailed table highlighting various vegetables suitable for a gluten-free diet. This includes ingredients, nutritional information, serving sizes, and cooking times to help those managing their diet:

Vegetable	Ingredient	Nutritional Information (per 100g serving)	Serving Size	Cooking Time
Asparagus	Fresh asparagus spears	20 calories, 2.2g protein, 0.2g fat, 2.1g fiber	5 spears	4-7 minutes (boiled)
Broccoli	Fresh broccoli florets	34 calories, 2.8g	1 cup	5-7 minutes (steamed)

		protein, 0.4g fat, 2.6g fiber		
Carrots	Fresh carrots	41 calories, 0.9g protein, 0.2g fat, 2.8g fiber	1 medium carrot	4-5 minutes (boiled)
Spinach	Fresh spinach leaves	23 calories, 2.9g protein, 0.4g fat, 2.2g fiber	1 cup	2-3 minutes (steamed)
Kale	Fresh kale leaves	49 calories, 4.3g protein, 0.9g fat, 2.0g fiber	1 cup	5-7 minutes (sauteed)

Sweet Potatoes	Fresh sweet potatoes	86 calories, 1.6g protein, 0.1g fat, 3.0g fiber	1 medium potato	45-50 minutes (baked)
Bell Peppers	Fresh bell peppers	20 calories, 0.9g protein, 0.2g fat, 1.7g fiber	1 medium pepper	5-6 minutes (roasted)
Zucchini	Fresh zucchini	17 calories, 1.2g protein, 0.3g fat, 1.0g fiber	1 medium zucchini	5-7 minutes (sauteed)
Eggplant	Fresh eggplant	25 calories, 1.0g protein, 0.2g fat, 3.0g fiber	1 cup	25-30 minutes (baked)

Tomatoes	Fresh tomatoes	18 calories, 0.9g protein, 0.2g fat, 1.2g fiber	1 medium tomato	2-3 minutes (boiled)
Green Beans	Fresh green beans	31 calories, 1.8g protein, 0.1g fat, 2.7g fiber	1 cup	5-6 minutes (boiled)
Brussels Sprouts	Fresh brussels sprouts	43 calories, 3.4g protein, 0.3g fat, 3.8g fiber	1 cup	6-7 minutes (steamed)
Cucumber	Fresh cucumber	16 calories, 0.7g protein, 0.1g fat, 0.5g fiber	1 medium cucumber	Raw or pickled

Cauliflower	Fresh cauliflower florets	25 calories, 1.9g protein, 0.3g fat, 2.0g fiber	1 cup	5-6 minutes (steamed)
Butternut Squash	Fresh butternut squash	45 calories, 1.0g protein, 0.1g fat, 2.0g fiber	1 cup	30-35 minutes (baked)

Each of these vegetables can be incorporated into a gluten-free diet without worry, as they are naturally free of gluten. They offer a variety of nutrients and are versatile in preparation, making them essential components of daily meals. Be sure to rinse them thoroughly before cooking to remove any potential contaminants, especially if they are not organically sourced. This table serves as a handy guide for those looking to enrich their diet while managing gluten sensitivities or celiac disease.

Proteins

Certainly! Below is a detailed table that includes a variety of gluten-free protein sources, along with instructions for preparation, nutritional information, serving size, and cooking time. This comprehensive guide will help those following a gluten-free diet to integrate a variety of healthy proteins into their meals.

Protein Ingredient	Preparation Instructions	Nutritional Information (per serving)	Serving Size	Cooking Time
Chicken Breast	Grill or bake with olive oil, salt, and pepper.	165 calories, 31g protein, 3.6g fat	1 breast (approx. 170g)	20-25 minutes at 375°F

Salmon	Bake with lemon slices and dill.	233 calories, 25g protein, 15g fat	1 fillet (approx. 180g)	15-20 minutes at 400°F
Quinoa	Rinse well, then simmer in water with a pinch of salt.	222 calories, 8g protein, 3.6g fat, 39g carbs	1 cup cooked	15-20 minutes
Lentils	Boil in water until tender.	230 calories, 18g protein, 15g fiber, 40g carbs	1 cup cooked	15-20 minutes

Black Beans	Soak overnight, rinse, and boil until soft.	227 calories, 15g protein, 0.9g fat, 41g carbs	1 cup cooked	60-90 minutes
Tofu (firm)	Press to remove excess water, then cube and stir-fry.	70 calories, 8g protein, 4g fat	1/2 cup (approx. 124g)	5-10 minutes
Chickpeas	Soak overnight, boil until tender. Can be roasted for a	269 calories, 14.5g protein, 4.25g fat, 45g carbs	1 cup cooked	60-90 minutes

	crunchy snack.			
Almonds	Eat raw or toasted for added flavor.	162 calories, 6g protein, 14g fat	1/4 cup (approx. 35g)	N/A (10 minutes to toast)
Eggs	Boil, scramble, or make an omelet with vegetables.	72 calories, 6g protein, 5g fat	1 large egg	6-12 minutes (boiled)
Greek Yogurt	Serve plain or with fruit and honey.	100 calories, 17g protein, 0.7g fat	1 cup	N/A

Cottage Cheese	Serve plain or with fruit.	206 calories, 23g protein, 9.5g fat	1 cup	N/A
Pork Loin	Roast with herbs and spices until fully cooked.	206 calories, 29g protein, 10.5g fat	4 oz (approx. 113g)	25 minutes at 375°F
Shrimp	Grill or sauté with garlic and herbs.	84 calories, 18g protein, 0.8g fat	3 oz (approx. 85g)	5-7 minutes

| Ground Turkey | Cook in a skillet with your favorite seasonings until browned. | 204 calories, 22g protein, 12g fat | 4 oz (approx. 113g) | 10-12 minutes |
| Tempeh | Slice and sauté with soy sauce and your choice of vegetables. | 162 calories, 15g protein, 9g fat | 3 oz (approx. 85g) | 10-12 minutes |

This table not only lists various sources of protein that are safe for a gluten-free diet but also provides practical cooking instructions and nutritional information to help manage dietary needs efficiently. Whether you're meal prepping or looking for quick and nutritious meal options, these protein sources are versatile and beneficial for maintaining a balanced, gluten-free diet.

Grains and Flours

Here's a detailed table for "Grains and Flours" that are gluten-free, including information about 15 different grains and flours, their nutritional benefits, serving sizes, and cooking times:

Grain/Fl our	Ingredie nt	Nutritio nal Informat ion (per 100g)	Serving Size	Cooking Time
1. Quinoa	Whole grain quinoa	Calories: 368, Protein: 14g, Fat: 6g, Carbohyd rates: 64g, Fiber: 7g	1/4 cup uncooked	15-20 minutes

2. Brown Rice	Whole grain brown rice	Calories: 370, Protein: 7.5g, Fat: 2.68g, Carbohydrates: 77.24g	1/4 cup uncooked	45 minutes
3. Millet	Whole grain millet	Calories: 378, Protein: 11g, Fat: 4.22g, Carbohydrates: 72.85g	1/4 cup uncooked	20-25 minutes
4. Sorghum	Whole grain sorghum	Calories: 339, Protein: 11.3g, Fat: 3.3g,	1/4 cup uncooked	50-55 minutes

		Carbohyd rates: 74g		
5. Amaranth	Whole grain amaranth	Calories: 371, Protein: 13.56g, Fat: 7.02g, Carbohyd rates: 65.25g	1/4 cup uncooked	20-25 minutes
6. Teff	Whole grain teff	Calories: 367, Protein: 13g, Fat: 2.38g, Carbohyd rates: 73.13g	1/4 cup uncooked	15-20 minutes

7. Cornmeal	Ground dried corn	Calories: 384, Protein: 8.1g, Fat: 4.3g, Carbohydrates: 80.2g	1/4 cup uncooked	10-15 minutes
8. Almond Flour	Ground almonds	Calories: 575, Protein: 21.15g, Fat: 49.93g, Carbohydrates: 21.55g	1/4 cup	N/A (used in baking)
9. Coconut Flour	Ground dried coconut	Calories: 443, Protein: 19.3g, Fat:	1/4 cup	N/A (used in baking)

		13.3g, Carbohydrates: 59.9g		
10. Buckwheat	Whole grain buckwheat	Calories: 343, Protein: 13.25g, Fat: 3.4g, Carbohydrates: 71.5g	1/4 cup uncooked	15-20 minutes
11. Oat Flour	Ground oats (GF)	Calories: 404, Protein: 14.66g, Fat: 9.12g, Carbohydrates: 65.7g	1/4 cup	N/A (used in baking)

12. Chickpea Flour	Ground chickpeas	Calories: 387, Protein: 22.39g, Fat: 6.69g, Carbohyd rates: 57.82g	1/4 cup	N/A (used in baking)
13. Arrowroo t Flour	Ground arrowroot	Calories: 357, Protein: 0.3g, Fat: 0.1g, Carbohyd rates: 88.2g	1/4 cup	N/A (used as thickener)
14. Cassava Flour	Ground cassava root	Calories: 340, Protein: 1.58g, Fat: 0.28g,	1/4 cup	N/A (used in baking)

		Carbohyd rates: 83.68g		
15. Potato Flour	Ground dried potatoes	Calories: 357, Protein: 6.9g, Fat: 0.3g, Carbohyd rates: 83.1g	1/4 cup	N/A (used in baking)

Each of these grains and flours offers unique benefits and applications, making them suitable for a variety of dietary needs, especially for those following a gluten-free diet. Note that cooking times for grains can vary based on the specific product and desired texture, so adjustments may be necessary. When using these ingredients, especially in baking, exact measurements and adherence to recipes are important for achieving the best results.

Dairy and Dairy Alternatives

Here's a detailed table focusing on dairy and dairy alternatives suitable for a gluten-free diet, including key ingredients, preparation instructions, nutritional information, serving sizes, and cooking times:

Product	Key Ingredients	Preparation Instructions	Nutritional Information (per serving)	Serving Size	Cooking Time
Whole Milk	Milk	Serve chilled or heat gently for hot beverages	150 calories, 8g fat, 12g carbs, 8g protein	1 cup (240 ml)	N/A

Greek Yogurt	Cultured milk	Serve chilled. Can be mixed with fruits or granola	100 calories, 4g fat, 6g carbs, 10g protein	100 grams	N/A
Almond Milk	Water, almonds	Shake well, serve chilled or use in recipes	30 calories, 2.5g fat, 1g carbs, 1g protein	1 cup (240 ml)	N/A
Coconut Milk	Coconut cream, water	Shake well, serve chilled or use	50 calories, 5g fat, 2g carbs,	1 cup (240 ml)	N/A

		in cooking	0.5g protein		
Soy Milk	Soybeans, water	Shake well, serve chilled or use in cooking	100 calories, 4g fat, 8g carbs, 7g protein	1 cup (240 ml)	N/A
Butter	Cream (milk)	Use as spread or in cooking /baking	100 calories, 11g fat, 0g carbs, 0g protein	1 tbsp (14g)	N/A
Cheddar Cheese	Milk, cheese cultures	Serve as is or melted	110 calories, 9g fat,	1 oz (28g)	N/A

	, enzymes	in dishes	1g carbs, 7g protein		
Cashew Cheese	Cashews, water, cultures	Serve chilled or spread on gluten-free crackers	90 calories, 7g fat, 5g carbs, 3g protein	1 oz (28g)	N/A
Rice Milk	Brown rice, water	Serve chilled or use in cereals and recipes	120 calories, 2.5g fat, 22g carbs, 1g protein	1 cup (240 ml)	N/A

Hemp Milk	Hemp seeds, water	Serve chilled, stir or shake if separated	60 calories, 4.5g fat, 0g carbs, 3g protein	1 cup (240 ml)	N/A
Oat Milk	Water, oats	Shake well, serve chilled or use in cooking	120 calories, 5g fat, 16g carbs, 3g protein	1 cup (240 ml)	N/A
Goat Cheese	Goat milk, salt, cultures	Serve chilled or crumbled over salads	75 calories, 6g fat, 0.1g carbs,	1 oz (28g)	N/A

			5g protein		
Feta Cheese	Sheep's milk, salt	Serve crumbled in salads or cooked in dishes	80 calories, 6g fat, 1g carbs, 4g protein	1 oz (28g)	N/A
Lactose -Free Milk	Lactase, milk	Serve chilled or use as regular milk in recipes	100 calories, 2.5g fat, 12g carbs, 8g protein	1 cup (240 ml)	N/A

| Flax Milk | Flaxseed oil, water | Serve chilled or use in smoothies and other recipes | 25 calories, 2.5g fat, 1g carbs, 0g protein | 1 cup (240 ml) | N/A |

This table provides a variety of dairy and dairy alternative options for those following a gluten-free diet, detailing everything necessary to incorporate these products effectively into daily meals and special recipes.

Fats and Oils

Below is a detailed table listing various fats and oils that are gluten-free, along with their ingredients, nutritional information, serving sizes, and cooking times. This table serves as a guide for individuals adhering to a gluten-free diet, providing essential details to help maintain this dietary requirement.

Fats/Oils	Ingredients	Nutritional Information per Serving	Serving Size	Cooking Time
Olive Oil	100% Pure Extracted Olive Oil	120 calories, 14g fat, 0g carbs, 0g protein	1 tbsp	NA
Coconut Oil	100% Pure	121 calories, 13.5g fat,	1 tbsp	NA

	Coconut Oil	0g carbs, 0g protein		
Avocado Oil	100% Pure Avocado Oil	124 calories, 14g fat, 0g carbs, 0g protein	1 tbsp	NA
Butter	Cream (Milk)	102 calories, 11.5g fat, 0.01g carbs, 0.12g protein	1 tbsp	NA
Ghee	Clarified Butter	112 calories, 12.8g fat, 0g carbs, 0g protein	1 tbsp	NA

Canola Oil	100% Pure Canola Oil	124 calories, 14g fat, 0g carbs, 0g protein	1 tbsp	NA
Vegetable Oil	Soybean Oil, Canola Oil	120 calories, 14g fat, 0g carbs, 0g protein	1 tbsp	NA
Grapeseed Oil	100% Pure Grapeseed Oil	120 calories, 14g fat, 0g carbs, 0g protein	1 tbsp	NA
Sesame Oil	100% Pure	120 calories, 14g fat, 0g	1 tbsp	NA

	Sesame Oil	carbs, 0g protein		
Peanut Oil	100% Pure Peanut Oil	119 calories, 14g fat, 0g carbs, 0g protein	1 tbsp	NA
Flaxseed Oil	100% Pure Flaxseed Oil	124 calories, 14g fat, 0g carbs, 0g protein	1 tbsp	NA
Walnut Oil	100% Pure Walnut Oil	120 calories, 14g fat, 0g carbs, 0g protein	1 tbsp	NA

Almond Oil	100% Pure Almond Oil	120 calories, 14g fat, 0g carbs, 0g protein	1 tbsp	NA
Sunflower Oil	100% Pure Sunflower Oil	120 calories, 14g fat, 0g carbs, 0g protein	1 tbsp	NA
Palm Oil	100% Pure Palm Oil	114 calories, 14g fat, 0g carbs, 0g protein	1 tbsp	NA

This table offers a broad range of gluten-free fats and oils, essential for cooking and baking within a gluten-free diet. The information is precise to aid in maintaining strict dietary adherence and ensuring each individual can enjoy varied, nutritious, and safe food options.

Beverages

Here is a detailed table of gluten-free beverages, including ingredient lists, instructions, nutritional information, serving sizes, and preparation or cooking times:

Beverage Name	Ingredients	Instructions	Nutritional Information per Serving	Serving Size	Preparation Time
1. Almond Milk	Almonds, water, salt, optional sweetener	Blend soaked almonds with water, strain, add salt/sweetener	Calories: 30, Fat: 2.5g, Protein: 1g	1 cup	10 minutes

2. Coconut Water	Pure coconut water	Chill and serve	Calories: 46, Fat: 0g, Protein: 2g	1 cup	-
3. Herbal Tea	Herbal tea leaves or bags, water	Steep tea leaves in boiled water for 5-7 minutes	Calories: 0, Fat: 0g, Protein: 0g	1 cup	7 minutes
4. Fruit Smoothie	Mixed fruit, yogurt, honey	Blend ingredients until smooth	Calories: 150, Fat: 2g, Protein: 3g	1 cup	5 minutes

5. **Vegetable Juice**	Carrots, tomatoes, celery, salt	Juice vegetables, stir in salt	Calories: 50, Fat: 0g, Protein: 2g	1 cup	15 minutes
6. **Rice Milk**	Cooked rice, water, salt	Blend cooked rice with water, strain, add salt	Calories: 120, Fat: 2.5g, Protein: 1g	1 cup	20 minutes
7. **Black Coffee**	Ground coffee beans, water	Brew ground beans with hot water	Calories: 2, Fat: 0g, Protein: 0g	1 cup	5 minutes

8. Lemon ade	Lemon juice, water, sugar	Mix all ingredie nts, chill	Calories : 99, Fat: 0g, Protein: 0g	1 cup	5 minutes
9. Kombu cha	Tea, sugar, SCOBY , flavorin gs (option al)	Fermen t tea and sugar with SCOBY for 7-30 days	Calories : 30, Fat: 0g, Protein: 0g	1 cup	7+ days
10. Bone Broth	Bones, water, vinegar, herbs	Simmer ingredie nts for 12-24 hours	Calories : 40, Fat: 0g, Protein: 10g	1 cup	24 hours

11. **Sparkling Water**	Carbonated water, natural flavoring	Chill and serve	Calories: 0, Fat: 0g, Protein: 0g	1 cup	-
12. **Iced Tea**	Tea bags, water, ice	Brew tea, cool, and serve with ice	Calories: 0, Fat: 0g, Protein: 0g	1 cup	10 minutes
13. **Ginger Ale**	Ginger, sugar, lemon juice, club soda	Simmer ginger with sugar and water, mix in lemon	Calories: 124, Fat: 0g, Protein: 0g	1 cup	30 minutes

		and soda			
14. Hot Chocol ate	Cocoa powder, milk or water, sugar	Heat milk, stir in cocoa and sugar	Calories : 192, Fat: 3.5g, Protein: 8g	1 cup	10 minutes
15. Sports Drink	Electrol ytes, sugar, water, flavorin g	Mix ingredie nts, chill	Calories : 50, Fat: 0g, Protein: 0g	1 cup	5 minutes

This table provides a comprehensive guide to a variety of gluten-free beverages, including both homemade and naturally gluten-free options. It details the necessary ingredients, simple preparation instructions, basic nutritional content, appropriate serving sizes, and the required time to prepare or brew each beverage.

Chapter 2: Foods to Avoid

Grains Containing Gluten

When adopting a gluten-free diet, it's crucial to be aware of grains that contain gluten because consuming these grains can lead to health issues for individuals with celiac disease, gluten sensitivity, or wheat allergies. Gluten is a protein found in several types of grains and can trigger an immune response in susceptible individuals. Here is a table outlining common grains containing gluten and reasons why they should be avoided if you're following a gluten-free lifestyle:

Grain	Contains Gluten	Why to Avoid	Commonly Found In
Wheat	Yes	Wheat gluten can cause digestive distress, damage to the small intestine, and other serious symptoms in	Breads, pastas, cereals, cakes, cookies, sauces, and many processed foods.

		people with celiac disease.	
Barley	Yes	Contains gluten that can trigger allergic reactions and exacerbate symptoms of celiac disease.	Malt beverages (like beer), food coloring, soups, malt vinegar, and some snacks.
Rye	Yes	Rye gluten is harmful for those with celiac disease or gluten intolerance, leading to similar symptoms as wheat.	Rye breads, rye beer, some cereals, and rye crackers.
Triticale	Yes	A hybrid of wheat and rye, triticale combines the	Some breads, cereals, and flours.

		glutens of both grains, making it especially harmful for those avoiding gluten.	
Spelt	Yes	Although often marketed as suitable for those with wheat allergies, spelt contains gluten and is not safe for individuals with celiac disease.	Certain pastas, breads, and specialty food products labeled as ancient or heirloom wheat.
Kamut	Yes	Contains gluten and can cause reactions in	Specialty breads, pastas, and grain

		those with gluten-related disorders.	products often touted as healthier alternatives.
Bulgur	Yes	Made from durum wheat, bulgur contains gluten and should be avoided by those on a gluten-free diet.	Tabouleh, pilafs, and some Mediterranean dishes.
Farro	Yes	An ancient wheat grain that contains gluten and can provoke celiac disease symptoms.	Soups, salads, risotto, and other grain-based dishes.
Durum	Yes	A type of wheat used in	Pasta, couscous,

		pasta-making, it contains gluten and can cause adverse health effects for gluten-sensitive individuals.	and some breads.
Semolina	Yes	A coarse, refined wheat middlings of durum wheat used in pasta and some bread, containing gluten.	Pasta, some breads, and porridge.

Understanding these grains and their effects is vital for maintaining a strict gluten-free diet. Avoiding these grains can prevent the symptoms associated with gluten intake, which range from gastrointestinal issues to neurological symptoms in severe cases. When purchasing grains, always look for those that are certified gluten-free, including corn, rice, quinoa, and buckwheat, to ensure they haven't been contaminated with gluten-bearing grains during processing.

Processed Foods and Risky Ingredients

Navigating the landscape of processed foods can be particularly challenging for individuals following a gluten-free diet. Many processed foods contain hidden sources of gluten or are at risk of cross-contamination during manufacturing. Understanding which processed foods and ingredients to avoid is crucial for maintaining a strict gluten-free diet. Below is a detailed table outlining common processed foods and risky ingredients, along with explanations for why they should be avoided.

Processed Food or Ingredient	Common Sources of Gluten	Reason to Avoid
Soy Sauce	Wheat	Traditionally made with wheat, soy sauce contains gluten, which can trigger reactions in individuals with celiac disease or gluten sensitivity. Alternatives like tamari may be fermented without

		wheat and labeled gluten-free.
Imitation Meats	Seitan (wheat gluten)	Many vegan and vegetarian products use seitan as a protein source, which is pure gluten. These should be avoided unless specifically marked gluten-free.
Breaded Foods	Bread crumbs, flour	Common in frozen snacks and meats, the breading almost always includes wheat flour, making them unsafe unless labeled gluten-free.
Baked Goods	Wheat flour	Cakes, cookies, pies, and pastries typically use wheat

		flour as a primary ingredient. Gluten-free alternatives should be specifically verified.
Pasta and Noodles	Wheat	Traditional pasta, including spaghetti and noodles, is made from wheat. Gluten-free pasta is available but should be confirmed by labeling.
Cereals and Breakfast Foods	Barley malt, wheat bran	Many cereals, especially those containing malt flavoring or wheat bran, include gluten. Gluten-free cereals are specifically labeled.

Soups and Sauces	Flour as a thickener	Wheat flour is a common thickening agent in cream-based soups and some sauces, posing a risk for those on a gluten-free diet.
Processed Snacks	Wheat starch, barley malt	Snack foods like pretzels, crackers, and certain chips often contain gluten. Safe alternatives are those labeled gluten-free.
Beer and Malt Beverages	Barley malt	Most beers and malt beverages are brewed from barley, a gluten-containing grain. Gluten-free beers are brewed specifically with gluten-free grains.

Salad Dressings and Condiments	Malt vinegar, wheat starch	Hidden gluten can be found in many dressings and condiments, often from thickeners or flavorings derived from gluten sources.

Avoiding these processed foods and ingredients is essential not only to prevent symptoms but also to avoid long-term health complications associated with gluten intake in sensitive individuals. By carefully selecting products and verifying their gluten-free status, individuals can safely enjoy a variety of foods without exposure to gluten.

Condiments and Sauces

When following a gluten-free diet, navigating the condiments and sauces aisle can be tricky because many common products unexpectedly contain gluten. This is often due to additives for flavoring, thickening, or as byproducts of processing. Here's a comprehensive table outlining popular condiments and sauces that typically contain gluten, their ingredients that contribute to this, and why they should be avoided on a gluten-free diet:

Condiment/Sauce	Gluten-Containing Ingredients	Why to Avoid
Soy Sauce	Wheat as a primary ingredient	Wheat is a direct source of gluten and is used extensively in traditional soy sauce production. Avoid unless labeled specifically as gluten-free.
Barbecue Sauce	Modified food starch, malt flavoring, wheat flour, soy sauce	These ingredients often derive from gluten-containing grains.

		Cross-contamination during manufacturing is also common.
Gravy	Wheat flour (as a thickener)	Wheat flour is commonly used to thicken gravies and sauces, making most commercial gravies unsafe unless specified as gluten-free.
Salad Dressings	Malt vinegar, wheat protein, modified food starch	These ingredients can be hidden sources of gluten in salad dressings. Malt vinegar is derived from barley, and modified food starch can be wheat-based unless otherwise stated.

Teriyaki Sauce	Wheat (found in soy sauce and other additives)	Traditional teriyaki sauce includes soy sauce, which contains wheat, posing a high risk for those on a gluten-free diet.
Ketchup	Modified food starch, malt vinegar	Some ketchup brands use these ingredients, which can be derived from wheat. Always check the label for a gluten-free certification.
Mustard	Wheat flour, malt vinegar	Certain types of mustard may include these ingredients for flavor and texture. Opt for brands that guarantee a gluten-free product.

Worcestershire Sauce	Malt vinegar, soy sauce	The inclusion of malt vinegar (from barley) and soy sauce (often with wheat) can make this sauce unsafe for those avoiding gluten.
Beer-Based Marinades	Beer (contains barley)	Any marinade containing beer is not gluten-free, as most beers are brewed with barley, which is a gluten-containing grain.
Pasta Sauces	Wheat flour, barley for thickening or flavor	Some pasta sauces use flour or barley as thickeners or flavor enhancers. Checking labels for gluten-free claims is essential.

It's important for individuals on a gluten-free diet to carefully read labels and seek products specifically labeled as gluten-free. Many manufacturers now cater to gluten-free needs and clearly mark their products, making it easier to enjoy a variety of condiments and sauces without the risk of gluten exposure. Additionally, being aware of common gluten-containing ingredients helps in making informed choices and avoiding health complications associated with gluten sensitivity or celiac disease.

Snacks and Convenience Foods

For individuals following a gluten-free diet, understanding which snacks and convenience foods to avoid is essential to prevent unintentional gluten intake, which can lead to health issues for those with celiac disease or gluten sensitivity. Below is a comprehensive table that outlines common snacks and convenience foods, their ingredients that typically contain gluten, and reasons to avoid them:

Snack/Convenience Food	Common Gluten-Containing Ingredients	Reasons to Avoid
Pretzels	Wheat flour, malt, yeast, barley	Contains wheat, which is a primary source of gluten. Malt and barley are additional sources that can trigger reactions.
Cookies and Biscuits	Wheat flour, barley malt extract	Wheat flour is used in most traditional baking and is high in gluten. Barley malt extract is

		often used for flavor but contains gluten.
Breaded Foods (e.g., chicken nuggets, fish sticks)	Wheat flour, breadcrumbs	Breaded foods are typically coated with wheat flour and breadcrumbs, both of which are rich in gluten.
Cereal Bars	Barley malt, wheat flakes, oat syrup	Even if made with oats, which can be gluten-free, these bars often contain barley malt or wheat additives that include gluten.
Instant Noodles	Wheat flour, soy sauce	The noodles are primarily made from wheat. Soy sauce often contains wheat unless labeled gluten-free.

Frozen Pizzas	Wheat-based crust, processed toppings	The crust is generally wheat-based, and some toppings may contain gluten as a binder or thickener.
Crackers	Wheat flour, barley malt extract	Similar to cookies, crackers are mostly made from wheat flour. Barley malt extract is sometimes used for flavoring.
Pie Crusts	Wheat flour	Traditional pie crusts are made from wheat flour, which is a high-gluten ingredient.
Beer and Malt Beverages	Barley	Beer is typically brewed from barley, which naturally contains

		gluten. Malt beverages also generally use barley.
Packaged Soups and Sauces	Wheat flour (as thickener), barley	Many soups and sauces use wheat flour as a thickening agent. Some sauces might include barley for flavor.

Individuals on a gluten-free diet should avoid these products unless they are specifically labeled as gluten-free. Unintentional consumption of gluten can cause significant health setbacks for those with celiac disease, leading to symptoms like digestive discomfort, nutrient deficiencies, and in some cases, more severe reactions. Careful label reading and opting for products certified gluten-free can help mitigate these risks and maintain a healthy diet.

Conclusion

Navigating a gluten-free lifestyle requires a firm commitment and a deep understanding of what it means to truly avoid gluten. Those who must adhere to this diet for health reasons, such as celiac disease, or those who choose it for personal health benefits, find that the initial transition can be challenging. However, over time, with the right resources and knowledge, it becomes manageable and even enjoyable to maintain a gluten-free diet.

One of the most empowering tools for managing a gluten-free lifestyle is a comprehensive gluten-free food list. Such a list does more than simply name the foods that are safe or unsafe; it educates individuals on how to identify hidden sources of gluten, which can often appear in unexpected places. With this knowledge, the risk of accidental gluten ingestion decreases significantly, leading to better health outcomes and a higher quality of life.

Additionally, a well-maintained gluten-free food list encourages variety and nutrition. By expanding the range of safe foods, individuals are less likely to feel restricted in their diet. This variety is crucial not only for nutritional balance but also for maintaining interest and pleasure in meals, which can sometimes feel limiting when major food groups like wheat are off-limits.

Moreover, the psychological benefits of having a reliable gluten-free food list should not be underestimated. The stress of having to scrutinize every label or question every meal choice can be taxing. A definitive guide alleviates much of this burden, providing peace of mind and reducing the anxiety associated with meal preparation and eating out.

For families and individuals who are new to gluten-free living, such a list can also serve as a critical educational tool. It can help them learn together about safe food preparation and cross-contamination, which are essential aspects of a gluten-free kitchen. This shared learning process not only helps in managing the diet but also in fostering understanding and support within the family or among friends.

The economic impact of following a gluten-free diet is another aspect where the food list proves beneficial. By knowing exactly what products are safe, individuals can avoid costly mistakes and wasteful purchases. This efficiency is particularly important given that many gluten-free products can be more expensive than their gluten-containing counterparts.

In conclusion, a comprehensive gluten-free food list is more than just a dietary tool—it's a roadmap to a safer, healthier, and more enjoyable lifestyle for those avoiding gluten. It supports sustained health management, ensures dietary variety, and enhances life quality, proving indispensable in the journey towards successful gluten-free living.